HOW TO NATURALLY REVERSE DIABETES & INSULIN RESISTANCE

No part of this book may be reproduced in any form or by any electronic or mechanical means including information storage and retrieval systems - except in the case of brief quotations embodied in the critical articles or reviews without permission in writing from the publisher.

This book is not intended as a substitute for medical advice from a qualified physician. This book intends to provide accurate general information regarding the subject matter covered. If medical advice or other expert help is needed, the services of an appropriate medical professional should be sought.

Table of Contents

Preface

Although Type II diabetes is an easily preventable and treatable chronic condition, diabetics are being drugged with insulin or metformin. If using insulin and metformin worked, the people using them wouldn't eventually end up with amputated limbs and other harmful diabetic conditions.

The Industrial food complex is knowingly overloading the body with sugar, artificial sweeteners, and highly addictive GMO(genetically engineered) high fructose corn syrup and its derivatives. Worse, these processed foods are purposely poisoned with hundreds of endocrine-blocking and disrupting herbicides and pesticides that have been shown to cause diabetes.

Unfortunately, people are woefully dependent on ultra-processed fast foods in most urban settings. When it comes to "home-cooked organic healthy foods", most people do not have the time to cook, have no idea how to cook, or cannot afford to cook. This situation leaves people in a dire situation.

Compounding this is leading social media sites and search engines are censoring alternative health, while allowing alternative health web search results to be dominated by drug-pushing pharmaceutical sponsored websites. This makes it extremely difficult for anyone to find simple natural remedies for diabetes or other medical conditions.

Introduction

Within this book, you'll find simple remedies to Type I/II diabetes & insulin resistance. You'll realize that diabetes is nothing to fear and that with a simple diet adjustment, adding a few simple minerals, or herbs, you'll regain full possession of your blood sugar metabolism.

Because we're being bombarded with sugar, hidden sugars, endocrine-disrupting pesticides, and herbicides. Statistically, everyone in modern society has some form of insulin resistance or pre-diabetes,

I once was insulin resistant and prediabetic for many years, I had many of the typical insulin resistance symptoms such as skin tags, the inability to lose weight with exercise, and fatty liver disease. Through much research, I learned how to reverse insulin resistance and diabetes. Within this book, I will share how I cured myself and others of diabetes.

Chapter 1

What is Diabetes

Diabetes is a condition that develops when your fasting blood sugar (glucose) is constantly too high. It develops when your pancreas isn't making enough insulin or your body's cells aren't responding properly to insulin(insulin resistance). People from any age group can be affected by diabetes, and if not mitigated, it can become a deadly lifelong chronic condition.

The carbohydrates(sugar, fiber, starch) that we eat are converted into blood glucose (sugar) by the liver. Your blood then transports glucose to all the body's cells for energy.

The body primarily stores glucose in skeletal muscles as glycogen. When blood sugar levels are too low, the pancreas releases glucagon a hormone that triggers the liver to convert glycogen into glucose and release it into the bloodstream, this process is called glycogenolysis. The liver can also manufacture necessary glucose by harvesting amino acids, waste products, and fat byproducts. This process is called gluconeogenesis.

When glucose is circulating in your bloodstream, your cells need a "key" for the cells to absorb the glucose. This key is insulin (a pancreatic hormone), it tells the cells to absorb the blood glucose. If your pancreas isn't making enough insulin or your body's cells aren't responding properly to insulin(insulin resistance), glucose builds up in your bloodstream, causing high blood sugar (hyperglycemia).

Over time, having consistently high blood glucose will eventually lead to diabetes, which can lead to serious health problems, such as heart disease, nerve damage, eye complications, and limb amputations.

The technical name for diabetes is diabetes mellitus. Another condition that shares the term "diabetes" is diabetes insipidus, but they're distinct. They share the name "diabetes" because they both cause increased thirst and frequent urination. Diabetes insipidus is much rarer than diabetes mellitus.

Types of Diabetes

There are several types of diabetes. The most common forms include:

- Type 2 diabetes: Your body doesn't make enough insulin, or your body's cells don't respond adequately to insulin (insulin resistance). This is the most common type of

- diabetes. It mainly affects adults, but children can have it as well.
- Prediabetes: This type is the stage before Type 2 diabetes. Your blood glucose levels are higher than normal but not high enough to be officially diagnosed with Type 2 diabetes.
- Type 1 diabetes: This type is "acclaimed" to be an autoimmune disease in which your immune system attacks and destroys insulin-producing cells in your pancreas for unknown reasons. Up to 10% of diabetics have Type 1 diabetes. It's typically diagnosed in children and young adults but can develop at any age.
- Gestational diabetes: This type develops in some people during pregnancy. Gestational diabetes usually goes away after pregnancy.

Other rare types of diabetes include:

- Type 3c diabetes: This form of diabetes happens when your pancreas has been damaged, which affects its ability to produce insulin. Pancreatitis, pancreatic cancer, cystic fibrosis, and hemochromatosis can all lead to pancreas damage that causes diabetes. Having your pancreas removed (pancreatectomy) also results in Type 3c.

- Latent autoimmune diabetes in adults (LADA): Like Type 1 diabetes, LADA also results from an "acclaimed" autoimmune reaction, but it develops much more slowly than Type 1. People diagnosed with LADA are usually over the age of 30.
- Maturity-onset diabetes of the young (MODY): MODY, also called monogenic diabetes, happens due to an inherited genetic mutation that affects how your body makes and uses insulin. There are currently over 10 different types of MODY. It affects up to 5% of people with diabetes and commonly runs in families.
- Neonatal diabetes: This is a rare form of diabetes that occurs within the first six months of life. It's also a form of monogenic diabetes. About 50% of babies with neonatal diabetes have the lifelong form called permanent neonatal diabetes mellitus. The condition disappears within a few months from onset, but it can come back later in life. This is called transient neonatal diabetes mellitus.
- Brittle diabetes: Brittle diabetes is a form of Type 1 diabetes marked by frequent and severe episodes of high and low blood sugar levels.

Chapter 2

What causes diabetes?

Diabetes can be caused by several factors, including dietary lifestyle, "genes", being overweight, obesity, excessive sugar consumption, lack of vitamins & minerals, pesticides & herbicides, pharmaceutical drugs, and physical inactivity.

Pharmaceutical drugs

Some Pharmaceutical drugs can damage beta cells(pancreatic cells that produce insulin) or disrupt how insulin functions. These include:
- certain types of diuretics, also called water pills
- anti-seizure drugs
- psychiatric drugs
- drugs to treat human immunodeficiency virus (HIV)
- pentamidine, a drug used to treat a type of pneumonia
- glucocorticoids, medicines used to treat inflammatory illnesses such as rheumatoid arthritis, asthma, lupus, and ulcerative colitis
- anti-rejection medicine used to help stop the body from rejecting a transplanted organ

Pesticides & Herbicides

Associations between **pesticide** exposure and diabetes risks were observed in plenty of epidemiological studies. Many *in vitro* and *in vivo* studies reported that pesticide exposure impaired glucose homeostasis and led to insulin resistance and diabetic symptoms.

Glyphosate, used in popular **herbicide Round-up**, is an endocrine disruptor, harms human health through food, and also has the potential to produce reactive oxygen species (ROS), which can lead to metabolic diseases. Glyphosate consumption from food has been shown to have a substantial part in insulin resistance, making it a severe concern to those with type 2 diabetes.

Chemicals

It has recently been shown that chemicals we encounter every day could be contributing to diabetes, such as:
- Dioxins
- Polychlorinated biphenyls (PCBs)
- Phthalates
- BPA

Researchers found that people with elevated levels of these chemicals were more likely to develop type 2 diabetes. Another study found a link between eating processed foods and type 2 diabetes. One possible reason that was cited is the toxic chemicals used in the packaging of these foods.

Vitamins & Minerals

Vitamin D
Vitamin D deficiency has been linked to the onset of diabetes. Several studies have shown a potential link between vitamin D deficiency and an increased risk of developing type 2 diabetes. A study of 100 participants found that taking a vitamin D supplement could reduce insulin resistance in type 2 diabetes. Another study of 120 participants found that vitamin D levels were lower for people with type 2 diabetes and that people with type 2 diabetes who take vitamin D supplements may have improved glucose management. Other studies have even shown higher levels of vitamin D to be associated with a lower risk of developing type 1 diabetes. The exact mechanism by which vitamin D affects blood glucose control has yet to be fully understood.

Some researchers believe that vitamin D plays a role in the production and secretion of insulin, the hormone that regulates blood sugar levels. Others suggest that vitamin D may help improve insulin sensitivity, allowing the body to use insulin more effectively.

In the research article "**Does Vitamin D Have a Role in Diabetes**". A nonrandomized control trial on 80 participants with type 1 diabetes, supported this idea and raised the point that low vitamin D is associated with insulin resistance and beta cell death, while also contributing to the development of type 1 diabetes.

Chromium
Chromium is an essential mineral beneficial in insulin regulation, carbohydrate, protein, and lipid metabolism. Chromium is an important factor in enhancing insulin activity. Studies show that people with type 2 diabetes have lower blood levels of chromium than those without the disease.

Magnesium
Type 2 diabetes is frequently associated with both extracellular and intracellular magnesium deficiency. Magnesium deficiency is common in patients with type 2 diabetes, especially in those

with poorly controlled glycemic profiles. Normal magnesium serum levels are essential for optimal functioning of many enzymes in insulin secretion and glucose and energy metabolism. Reduced intracellular magnesium concentrations result in defective tyrosine-kinase activity, postreceptorial insulin action impairment, and worsening insulin resistance in diabetic patients. A low magnesium intake and an increased magnesium urinary loss appear to be the most important mechanisms that may favor magnesium depletion in patients with type 2 diabetes. Also, a low dietary magnesium intake has been related to the development of type 2 diabetes and metabolic syndrome.

Obesity & Inactivity

The accumulation of excessive body fat can cause type 2 diabetes, and the risk of type 2 diabetes increases linearly with an increase in body mass index. Accordingly, the worldwide increase in the prevalence of obesity has led to a rise in the prevalence of type 2 diabetes. The cellular and physiological mechanisms responsible for the link between obesity and type 2 diabetes are complex and involve adiposity-induced alterations in β cell function, adipose tissue biology, and multi-organ insulin resistance, which are often alleviated and can even be normalized with adequate weight loss. Not getting enough physical activity can raise a person's risk of developing type 2 diabetes. Physical activity helps control blood glucose, weight, and blood pressure and helps increase "good" cholesterol and lower "bad" cholesterol.

A small study published in **"The Journals of Gerontology, Series A,"** elucidated how inactivity can lead to diabetes. The research showed that an abrupt drop in physical activity for a short time significantly increased glucose and insulin levels in older adults with prediabetes and that many patients were unable to return to their previous state of health even after resuming normal activity.

Chapter 3

What is Insulin Resistance?

Insulin resistance is a chronic condition that occurs when cells in your muscles, fat, and liver reject glucose(sugar). Insulin, a hormone essential to life, is synthesized in and excreted by your pancreas which regulates blood glucose levels. Insulin resistance can be temporary or chronic but can be reversed.

How does insulin function:

- Your body converts the food you eat into glucose, your body's main source of energy.
- When glucose enters your bloodstream, your pancreas releases insulin.
- Insulin aids glucose in your blood to enter your muscle, fat, and liver cells so they can use it for energy or store it for later use.
- Once glucose enters your cells and the glucose levels in your bloodstream decrease, your pancreas stops producing & releasing insulin.

For many reasons, your muscle, fat, and liver cells cannot respond inappropriately to insulin, which means the body's cells can't efficiently absorb glucose from the blood or store it. This is what is known as **insulin resistance**. As a result, your pancreas creates more insulin in an attempt to overcome your increasing blood glucose levels. This condition is called **hyperinsulinemia**.

Reasons why Insulin resistance develops:

According to the PubMed Article "**The Effect of Exercise and Heat on Mineral Metabolism and Requirements** ", strenuous exercise:

"Recent research has indicated that chromium requirements may be influenced by strenuous exercise. Anderson et al. (1984) reported that serum chromium concentrations were increased in adult males immediately after a 6-mile run at near-maximal running capacity. This increase in serum chromium was still evident 2 hours after the completion of the run, and urinary chromium loss was elevated twofold on the run day compared to non-run days……Rose et al. (1970) reported that serum magnesium concentrations in marathon runners immediately following a race were significantly lower than prerace values, a phenomenon that was attributed to sweat losses of the element during the run….The typical reduction in plasma magnesium following intense exercise is

on the order of 10 percent. Stendig-Lindberg et al. (1989) reported that low plasma magnesium concentrations can be demonstrated in young men for up to 18 days after strenuous exertion (a 70-km march). In addition to an increased loss of magnesium via sweat, urinary magnesium loss can increase by up to 30 percent following a bout of intense exercise."

Meaning, the more you sweat and urinate due to exercise the more you lose these two minerals, magnesium and chromium, that are integral to insulin sensitivity. Not replenishing these minerals with supplementation individuals will eventually develop insulin resistance. This is why I see people at my gym every day whether doing aerobics or resistance training, gradually put on body fat or do not lose body fat. Also, when you have insulin resistance, you have high circulating insulin in the blood which turns off the mechanism that allows fat to be burnt as fuel.

One must also consider that the mineral-depleted farm soils in the US make it a near impossibility to get proper nutrition from diet. Worse, the FDA allows hundreds of endocrine-blocking/disrupting diabetes-causing herbicides, pesticides, and chemicals in the food supply and cosmetic products.

According to Endocrine.org, it states in their article **"Endocrine-Disrupting Chemicals"** –

"Endocrine-disrupting chemicals (EDCs) are chemicals or mixtures of chemicals that interfere with the way the body's hormones work. Some EDCs act like "hormone mimics" and trick our body into thinking that they are hormones, while other EDCs block natural hormones from doing their job. Other EDCs can increase or decrease the levels of hormones in our blood by affecting how they are made, broken down, or stored in our body. Finally, other EDCs can change how sensitive our bodies are to different hormones.

EDCs can disrupt many different hormones, which is why they have been linked to numerous adverse human health outcomes including alterations in sperm quality and fertility, abnormalities in sex organs, endometriosis, early puberty, altered nervous system function, immune function, certain cancers, respiratory problems, metabolic issues, diabetes, obesity, cardiovascular problems, growth, neurological and learning disabilities, and more."

This research article explains why 50% of the US population has either diabetes or prediabetes. From my research, the majority of people in the US have insulin resistance to some degree.

Thyroid disorders can also cause insulin resistance, according to the PubMed article "**Insulin resistance and thyroid disorders**", states –

"Thyroid hormones have a significant effect on glucose metabolism and the development of insulin resistance. In hyperthyroidism, impaired glucose tolerance may be the result of mainly hepatic insulin resistance, whereas in hypothyroidism the available data suggests that the insulin resistance of peripheral tissues prevails."

The PubMed research article *"**Study of Insulin Resistance in Subclinical Hypothyroidism**"* states –

"Thyroid hormones T3 and T4 maintain a fine balance of glucose homeostasis by acting as insulin agonistic and antagonistic. Hypothyroidism can break this equilibrium and alter glucose metabolism, which can lead to insulin resistance."

Many naturally occurring vitamins and minerals needed for the body to metabolize sugar, such as chromium and magnesium, are removed during the refining process to create white sugar and flour.

Only iron and three synthetically created vitamins thiamin, riboflavin, and niacin, are added to the refined flour to equal its previous levels. As of note, since 1998, synthetic folic acid has now been added to grain products in the US.

If people continue to regularly over-consume refined nutrient-depleted carbohydrates, high-fructose corn syrup, and sugar-loaded sodas, they will develop insulin resistance and diabetes. This will most likely transpire even if they supplement with the necessary minerals. Your body's cells will gradually start to resist insulin, blocking glucose from entering the cells, and your pancreas B-cells which secrete insulin will eventually stop functioning due to the the excess glucose continually circulating in the blood.

Signs and symptoms of insulin resistance:

- **Excessive hunger and thirst**: If your body isn't producing enough insulin, excess glucose builds up in your blood. This overburdens your kidneys by forcing them to pull water from your body to create enough urine to carry out the additional glucose.
- **High fasting blood sugar levels**: When your pancreas can't make enough insulin to keep

- your blood sugar levels in a healthy range, it leads to elevated blood sugar levels and eventually to prediabetes and Type 2 Diabetes. Your fasting blood glucose is considered high if it remains elevated for 8-10 hours after your last meal.
- **Abnormally high blood pressure**: There is a link between insulin resistance and high blood pressure, so it's important to realize that you may be at increased risk for IR if you have high blood pressure.
- **Unexplained weight gain and difficulty losing weight**: When your cells stop responding appropriately to insulin, your body's glucose levels become elevated, promoting fat storage in your liver. This cycle continuously repeats, causing you to gain weight and have difficulty shedding it. When insulin is circulating in the blood it turns off the mechanism allowing for fat to be burnt as fuel. The weight centers around the abdomen.
- **Skin tags**: Researchers have found that skin tags (small growths on the skin) or dark patches of skin are often found on obese people and those with insulin resistance.
- **Hair loss**: One study of 324 women found that women who had some markers of insulin resistance (including waist circumference,

- neck circumference, waist-to-hip ratio, and insulin concentration in the blood, among others) had a significantly higher risk for female androgenic alopecia (AGA), or female pattern baldness. This appears to happen because higher than average levels of sugar in your bloodstream can reduce the growth cycle of your hair, leading to hair loss.
- **Constant lethargy or fatigue**: Research on diabetic patients has found strong correlations between insulin resistance and fatigue.
- **Vaginal** and **skin infections**.
- **Adult Acne**
- **Slow-healing** cuts and sores.
- **Darkened skin** in the folds of the skin such as your armpit or back and sides of your neck, called acanthosis nigricans.

As long as your pancreas can create enough insulin to overcome your cells' resistance to insulin, your blood sugar levels will stay within a healthy range. If your cells become too resistant to insulin, it leads to dangerously elevated blood glucose levels known as **hyperglycemia**, which can lead to prediabetes and Type 2 diabetes.

In addition to **Type 2 diabetes**, insulin resistance is associated with several other conditions, including:

- Obesity.
- Cardiovascular disease.
- Nonalcoholic fatty liver disease.
- Metabolic syndrome.
- Polycystic ovary syndrome (PCOS).
- Alzheimer's and dementia
- Uterine Fibroids
- Enlarged Prostate

How to reverse insulin resistance?

Insulin resistance is primarily a result of mineral deficiencies and a lifestyle condition. I've listed below many reference research articles proving this fact. After the listed research articles, I elucidate the formula I used to reverse my insulin resistance successfully.

The December 2016 issue of Asia Pacific Journal of Clinical Nutrition reported in the article, **"Combined chromium and magnesium decreases insulin resistance more effectively than either alone"**, the outcome of a study from China's Medical College of Qingdao University which found drastic improvement in insulin resistance in middle-aged individuals who supplemented with magnesium and chromium.

"One hundred-twenty insulin resistant subjects between the ages of 45 to 59 years were divided into groups who received 160 micrograms per day chromium, 200 milligrams per day magnesium, chromium plus magnesium, or a placebo for three months. Fasting blood glucose, fasting insulin, insulin resistance index, and T-lymphocyte messenger RNA levels of glucose transporter 4 (GLUT4, a protein that transports insulin) and glycogen-synthase-kinase-3beta (GSK3beta, an enzyme) were determined before and after treatment.

In the group that received both magnesium and chromium, fasting blood glucose, fasting insulin, insulin resistance index, and GSK3beta were significantly lower at the end of the study. Additionally, a 2.9-fold increase in GLUT4 was observed only among those who received both minerals...

GLUT4 and GSK3beta are important components in an insulin-induced signal transduction pathway that plays a key role in glucose metabolism," authors Mei Dou, PhD, and colleagues explain. "Increased expression of GLUT4 has been associated with enhanced glucose translocation from the exterior to the interior of cells in insulin-sensitive tissues and repression of GSK3beta has been shown to enhance insulin receptor activity.

As anticipated, we found that combined chromium/magnesium supplementation ameliorated insulin resistance more effectively than chromium or magnesium alone, and this effect was likely related to the regulation by combined chromium/magnesium of the expression of GLUT4 and GSK3beta," they conclude. "The results of the present study suggest the therapeutic potential of combined chromium/magnesium therapy in insulin resistant individuals."

The research article "**Magnesium supplementation enhances insulin sensitivity and decreases insulin resistance in diabetic rats**" states-

"Magnesium supplementation enhanced insulin sensitivity and decreased insulin resistance in diabetic rats mainly through increasing insulin receptor expression, affinity, and augmenting insulin receptor signaling. Magnesium supplementation also inhibited lipid peroxidation in diabetic rats and protected against pancreatic cell injury in diabetic rats. In addition, we found that β-arrestin-2 gene expression was suppressed in

diabetes, which was possibly attributed to gene methylation modification, as β-arrestin 2 promotor was rich in methylation-regulating sites. Magnesium supplementation could affect β-arrestin-2 gene expression and methylation."

The research article "**Oral Magnesium Supplementation Improves Insulin Sensitivity and Metabolic Control in Type 2 Diabetic Subjects: A randomized double-blind controlled trial**" states-

"RESULTS—At the end of the study, subjects who received magnesium supplementation showed significant higher serum magnesium concentration (0.74 ± 0.10 vs. 0.65 ± 0.07 mmol/l, P = 0.02) and lower HOMA-IR index (3.8 ± 1.1 vs. 5.0 ± 1.3, P = 0.005), fasting glucose levels (8.0 ± 2.4 vs. 10.3 ± 2.1 mmol/l, P = 0.01), and HbA1c (8.0 ± 2.4 vs. 10.1 ± 3.3%, P = 0.04) than control subjects.

CONCLUSIONS—Oral supplementation with MgCl2 solution restores serum magnesium levels, improving insulin sensitivity and metabolic control in type 2 diabetic patients with decreased serum magnesium levels."

This research article "**A scientific review: the role of chromium in insulin resistance**" states –

"Chromium is an essential mineral that appears to have a beneficial role in the regulation of insulin action and its effects on carbohydrate, protein and lipid metabolism. Chromium is an important factor for enhancing insulin activity. Studies show that people with type 2 diabetes have lower blood levels of chromium than those without the disease……Chromium picolinate, specifically, has been shown to reduce insulin resistance and to help reduce the risk of cardiovascular disease and type 2 diabetes. Dietary chromium is poorly absorbed. Chromium levels decrease with age. Supplements containing 200-1,000 mcg chromium as chromium picolinate a day have been found to improve blood glucose control."

The research article "**Effect of vanadium on insulin sensitivity and appetite**" states –

"Vanadium, a potent nonselective inhibitor of protein tyrosine phosphatases, has been shown to mimic many of the metabolic actions of insulin both in vivo and in vitro. The mechanism(s) of the effect of vanadium on the decrease in appetite and body weight in Zucker fa/fa rats, an insulin-resistant

model, is still unclear ... These data indicate that BMOV may increase insulin sensitivity in adipose tissue and decrease appetite and body fat by decreasing NPY levels in the hypothalamus. BMOV-induced reduction in appetite and weight gain along with normalized insulin levels in models of obesity, suggest its possible use as a therapeutic agent in obesity."

Following the advice in the Asia Pacific Journal of Clinical Nutrition article, I added 200mcg of chromium per major meal with 400mg of magnesium glycinate daily. To help quickly reverse my NAFLD liver(fatty liver) I took 150mg of milk thistle extract twice a day for a couple of months. Surprisingly my insulin resistance subsided quickly, in about two weeks. But I also predominately eat organic whole foods and only eat three meals daily without snacking between meals. The cause of my insulin resistance was not replenishing lost magnesium and chromium due to resistance training five days a week.

Also if you're trying to lose weight and are on a "typical" American diet, you'll need to do intermittent fasting. Meaning, you'll need to stop all snacking in between meals. If you snack your insulin levels will stay high throughout the day, and you'll never burn fat. As long as insulin is circulating in your blood, it signals your brain to turn off the body's ability to utilize fat as energy.

You can't be immobile and sit in your car, desk, and sofa all day and night. Humans were not designed nor evolved to consume as much "sugar" as we are, food (especially highly refined processed food), while having a sedentary lifestyle…..you have to exercise!!! Even if it's just walking… do something. You have to balance living in the concrete jungle with all of its conveniences, or you will get insulin resistance and eventually diabetes.

You can eat carbs too just like the French and Italians, just avoid "white bread", bleached "white flour", and other products made with highly refined carbohydrates laden with chemicals and preservatives. Eat more whole foods, drink natural alkaline water and non-concentrate unfiltered low glycemic organic fruit juices, and learn to cook!

Also, be aware that drinking coffee depletes your body of magnesium and chromium! Detox your liver once a month with Milk Thistle extract!

Chapter 4

How to Reverse Type 2 Diabetes

There are different ways to develop diabetes; likewise, there are a few ways to reverse diabetes. Some people may only need to apply one of the recommended protocols below.

Exercise & Diet

Some people have found by just changing their diet and being physically active over time they reversed their insulin resistance, prediabetes, or type 2 diabetes.

How? First, stop eating all processed foods with added sugar, read all the food labels for hidden sugars using ambiguous names like beet sugar, brown rice syrup, glucose, high fructose corn syrup, and corn syrup. The food labels will tell you how much total sugar is in a product, and it will tell you how much "added sugar" is also included if so. Stop drinking sodas, these are the primary beasts causing diabetes. Research has shown that consuming one sugary drink daily puts one pound of fat on your body every thirteen days. Drink water and either temporarily stop or drink sparingly low glycemic natural juices that are not from concentrate. Only unfiltered juices that include natural fiber and pulp.

Try to make your diet encompass as many low-glycemic foods as possible.

When you drink concentrated juices with added sugar there is no pulp and fiber to buffer the sugar entering your bloodstream causing blood sugar spikes.

You should opt for 100% organic natural juices with 0% added sugars and avoid fruit juices made from pineapple or mangos. These fruit juices often have a significant amount of sugar. Instead, stick with unsweetened lemon or grapefruit juice, which has a lower glycemic index than most other juices.

Although in America refined carbohydrates are demonized. It's because refined carbohydrates in America are poisoned with excessive refined sugars, endocrine-blocking/disrupting pesticides & herbicides, and food chemical additives that are generally limited or banned in most of Europe and other parts of the world.

Don't overindulge in refined carbohydrates, but you can buy European bread from European bakeries, most of them do not put added sugars in their bread, and if they do it's minimal, and they only use four or five natural ingredients. Even better bake your own bread with imported European "00" organic flour; "00" is easily digestible gluten. Eat wholesale organic foods, cook more, and try to eliminate as many processed foods as possible. Avoid white flour, white eggs, white granulated sugar, aspartame, and at all costs anything with High fructose corn syrup.

Do not munch or drink sweetened drinks between meals, that will keep your insulin levels high, eat only three or two wholesome meals a day.

Constant High fasting Insulin levels (hyperinsulinemia) shut down your body's fat-burning mechanism. So by subsisting on three meals a day, your insulin levels will be low and you'll be able to tackle those unwanted fat cells.

Get a gym membership, buy a treadmill, or walk around the block before or after you get off of work. Any form of prolonged physical activity, especially if you are overweight will help to reverse diabetic conditions.

Resistance training is one of the best exercises for diabetics/insulin resistance because it increases the number of muscle cells. The more muscle cells you have, the more calories you burn, and the more blood glucose your body uses. If you're obese reducing your body weight is critical in reversing diabetic conditions. Just by monitoring your blood sugar and making these simple adjustments to your lifestyle, many people have permanently reversed diabetes.

Insulin Resistance

I was unknowingly insulin-resistant for many years, definitely well over a decade. Not only that, but I was also prediabetic. After doing prolonged research I discovered that a lack of minerals was the main cause of insulin resistance. As for me, I'm always at the gym doing resistance training sweating out my minerals without replenishing them. We're not going to get proper minerals from foods because the commercial farm soils in the USA are depleted of minerals due to farming practices. So if we do not supplement with bioavailable minerals we'll develop ailments.

So once I added chromium picolinate and magnesium glycinate to my daily diet all of my insulin-resistant symptoms subsided within a few weeks. My skin tags disappeared, the dark skin between my thighs lightened and became uniform with the rest of my body's tone, my love handles started to shrink, and my frequent nighttime urination stopped.

To reverse insulin resistance see Chapter 3 "How to reverse insulin resistance".

Nigella Sativa

The heal-all powdered nigella sativa powder is well known for treating cancer, and infectious diseases. But little known is its anti-diabetic properties.

For people on insulin rather than metformin, I have recommended nigella sativa powder to many type 2 diabetics. I suggested they ingest ½ a teaspoon of the nigella powder twice daily. Typically within one month, they all reported their blood glucose was under control, and they no longer needed insulin injections.

If you're on metformin, you have insulin resistance. In this case, I recommend following the instructions in Chapter 3 "How to reverse insulin resistance".

Below are some research articles elucidating nigella sativa's efficacy in reversing diabetes.

The research article" **Antidiabetic Activity of Nigella Sativa (Black Seeds) and Its Active Constituent (Thymoquinone): A Review of Human and Experimental Animal Studies**", it states -

"The effect of Nigella sativa on the glycemic control was assessed through measurement of fasting blood glucose (FBG), blood glucose level 2 hours postprandially (2 hPG), and glycosylated hemoglobin (HbA1c). Serum C-peptide and changes in body weight were also measured. Insulin resistance and beta-cell function were calculated using the homeostatic model assessment (HOMA2)."

"Nigella sativa at a dose of 2 gm/day caused significant reductions in FBG, 2hPG, and HbA1 without significant change in body weight. Fasting blood glucose was reduced by an average of 45, 62 and 56 mg/dl at 4, 8 and 12 weeks respectively. HbAlC was reduced by 1.52% at the end of the 12 weeks of treatment (P<0.0001). Insulin resistance calculated by HOMA2 was reduced significantly

(P<0.01), while B-cell function was increased (P<0.02) at 12 weeks of treatment. "

The research article "**Effects of Nigella Sativa on Type-2 Diabetes Mellitus: A Systematic Review**" states-

"Nigella Sativa OR black seed oil OR thymoquinone OR black cumin AND diabetes mellitus OR hyperglycemia OR blood glucose OR hemoglobin A1C had returned 875 relevant articles. A total of seven articles were retrieved for further assessment and underwent data extraction to be included in this review. Nigella sativa was shown to significantly improve laboratory parameters of hyperglycemia and diabetes control after treatment with a significant fall in fasting blood glucose, blood glucose level 2 h postprandial, glycated hemoglobin, and insulin resistance, and a rise in serum insulin. In conclusion, these findings suggested that Nigella sativa could be used as an adjuvant for oral antidiabetic drugs in diabetes control."

The research article "**EFFECTS OF NIGELLA SATIVA L. SEED OIL IN TYPE II DIABETIC PATIENTS: A RANDOMIZED,**

**DOUBLE-BLIND, PLACEBO -
CONTROLLED CLINICAL TRIAL**" states -

"Methods: A randomized clinical trial was conducted in 70 type II diabetic patients referring to Baqiyatallah Hospital. The subjects were enrolled into two groups of 35 each. One group received 2.5 ml N. sativa oil and the other group received similarly 2.5 ml mineral oil two times a day for three months. The fasting and 2 hour postprandial blood glucose, glycosylated hemoglobin (HbA1c), lipid profile, BMI (body mass index), liver and renal function test were determined at the baseline and after three months. Results: The blood levels of fasting and 2 hours postprandial glucose and HbA1c were significantly decreased in the N. sativa group compared with the placebo group at the end of the study. The BMI of the N. sativa group was decreased significantly from baseline. No side effects were reported. Conclusion: N. sativa oil improves glycemic control in type II diabetic patients without any side effects."

Vitamin D

Vitamin D deficiency has been linked to the onset of diabetes. Vitamin D helps to maintain the normal release of insulin by the pancreatic beta cells (β-cells). Diabetes, as stated previously, is initiated by the onset of insulin resistance. The β-cells attempt to overcome this resistance by releasing more insulin, thus preventing hyperglycemia. However, as this hyperactivity increases, the β-cells experience excessive Ca2+(Calcium ions) and reactive oxygen species (ROS) signaling that results in β-cell cell death and the onset of diabetes. Vitamin D deficiency contributes to both the initial insulin resistance and the subsequent onset of diabetes caused by β-cell death. As an anti-inflammatory, vitamin D reduces inflammation, which is a major process in inducing insulin resistance. Vitamin D maintains the low levels of Ca2+ and ROS that are elevated in the β-cells during diabetes. Epigenetic alterations are a feature of diabetes by which many diabetes-related genes are inactivated by hypermethylation. Vitamin D acts to prevent such hypermethylation by increasing the expression of the DNA demethylases that prevent hypermethylation of multiple gene promoter regions of many diabetes-related genes. When Vitamin D is deficient, many of these processes begin to decline and this sets the stage for the onset of diseases such as diabetes.

Studies indicate that the average U.S. adult consumes about 230 IU of vitamin D per day. However, it has been estimated that 1,000 to 2,000 IU is necessary to satisfy the body's needs for most people. Many experts in the field suggest the recommended daily intake of vitamin D be increased to at least 2,000 IU of vitamin D daily, particularly for people in higher latitudes and in areas of extreme winter climate. A dose of vitamin D3 up to 2,000 IU daily has been deemed safe by the U.S. Food and Drug Administration's nutritional guidelines. However, a recent review concluded that the safe upper limit for vitamin D consumption is 10,000 IU per day.

After reading many research articles on using vitamin D to reverse many ailments, I have experimented and taken up to 30,000 IU of vitamin D daily for many months without an issue. It's very important to supplement with bio-available magnesium when taking vitamin D because the liver and pancreas use magnesium to convert vitamin D to its active hormonal form. Without sufficient blood serum magnesium, you will not reap the benefits of supplementing with vitamin D. Vitamin D deficiency-related ailments such as diabetes disproportionately affect dark-skinned people. Dark pigmentation known as melanin, actually blocks the absorption of ultraviolet light, especially in the more temperate regions of the earth. Dark-skinned people who supplement with vitamin D will not only possibly alleviate their diabetes, but also many other vitamin D deficiency related ailments.

Magnesium

Magnesium is a mineral that plays many important roles in your body, including managing your insulin and carbohydrate metabolism. It's involved in your body's pancreas's ability to secrete insulin and assist your cells use insulin more effectively.

Magnesium aids in managing blood sugar levels among people with diabetes. Also, those who tend to consume less magnesium typically have poorer blood sugar regulation and a higher risk of type 2 diabetes than people who consume a higher amount.

For example, in the article **"Oral magnesium supplementation in type II diabetic patients"**, a 12-week study in 54 people with type 2 diabetes found that taking 300 mg of magnesium daily significantly lowered fasting blood sugar levels, as well as post-meal blood sugar levels, compared with taking a placebo pill.

The research article "**The Therapeutic Effects of Magnesium in Insulin Secretion and Insulin Resistance**" states -

"Mg2+(magnesium) involves in more than 300 enzymatic reactions and numerous physiological processes by acting as a cofactor for many enzymes such as energy metabolism, glucose transport across cell membrane, hepatic gluconeogenesis, pancreatic functions, insulin secretion, and action in pancreatic cells and target tissues through interaction with receptors of this hormone. On this basis, intracellular Mg2+ balancing is vital for adequate carbohydrate metabolism. Studies have indicated that daily Mg2+ supplements may improve glycemic response among T2D patients and also prevent MetS(metabolic syndrome)"

Depending on which amino acid magnesium is chelated to, determines its bioavailability to the human body. Chelated forms of magnesium you want to avoid are -

Magnesium oxide: is a non-chelated type of magnesium with very little bioavailability to the human body.

Magnesium aspartate and Glutamate: These forms of magnesium contain glutamic acid and aspartic acid which are components in the artificial sweetener aspartame, which is neurotoxic.

The best forms of magnesium I have found are **magnesium glycinate** and transdermal **magnesium chloride**.

How much magnesium should I take?

Women should take 350mg daily, while men should get 400mg, If either is physically active more magnesium should be taken, as you lose magnesium in perspiration. Children aged 7 to 10 years should take 100 to 135 mg daily. Children 4 to 6 years old should take 65 mg per day. Children 3 years or under should take 20 to 50 mg daily. You must supplement more than the daily RDI if you are physically active.

Cacao

Cacao has been seen to improve oxidative stress and enhance insulin sensitivity. Recent in vitro and animal model studies have investigated the potential of cacao and its extracts in modulating fatty liver and pancreatic function. Evidence from these studies has highlighted several mechanisms, which facilitate insulin secretion and enhanced survival in pancreatic beta cells. In the liver, an improved effect of insulin was observed with some improvements in fatty infiltration.

Epicatechin, a natural flavonoid found in cacao and green tea, helps manage diabetes. Epicatechin has been shown to reduce blood glucose levels in diabetic patients. Epicatechin may decrease insulin resistance, it also has antioxidant and anti-inflammatory properties. Some studies have suggested that epicatechin may help with diabetes by reshaping the gut microbiota and gut-liver axis and preventing glutathione depletion in beta-cells.

Epicatechin has been shown to have several effects on pancreatic beta cells, which are responsible for producing insulin to regulate glucose homeostasis. Epicatechin can increase glucose-stimulated insulin secretion (GSIS) in healthy beta-cell lines and isolated islets. Epicatechin can help restore beta cell mass and function in oxidant-stressed beta cell lines, isolated islets, or animals. Supplementation with epicatechin-rich foods, such as cacao, can improve insulin sensitivity and glucose tolerance in people with type 2 diabetes.

The Research article "**Dietary Flavonol Epicatechin Prevents the Onset of Type 1**

Diabetes in Non-obese Diabetic (NOD) Mice" states -

"Type 1 diabetes (T1D) is an autoimmune disease characterized by the selective destruction of pancreatic β-cells. Although successful islet transplantation provides a promising treatment, high cost, lack of donor organs, immune-mediated destruction of transplanted islets, and side effects from immunosuppressive drugs greatly limit its uses. Therefore, the search for novel and cost-effective agents that can prevent or ameliorate T1D is extremely important to decrease the burden of T1D. In this study, we discovered that epicatechin (EC, 0.5% in drinking water), a flavonol primarily in cocoa, effectively prevented T1D in non-obese diabetic (NOD) mice. At 32 weeks of age, 66.7% control mice had overt diabetes, whereas only 16.6% EC-treated mice became diabetic. Consistently, EC mice had significantly higher plasma insulin levels but lower glycosylated hemoglobin concentrations compared to control mice. EC had no significant effects on food or water intake and body weight gain in NOD mice, suggesting that EC's effect was not due to alterations in these variables. Treatment with EC elevates circulating anti-inflammatory cytokine interleukin-10 levels, ameliorates pancreatic insulitis, and improved pancreatic islet mass. These

findings demonstrate that EC may be a novel, plant-derived compound capable of preventing T1D by modulating immune function and thereby preserving islet mass."

How to Reverse Type 1 Diabetes

Type 1 diabetes is a rare form of diabetes, and it's also the form that will take longer to reverse from my personal experience.

I have successfully reversed type 1 diabetes in an adult woman using this formula of 7.5mg vanadium(vanadyl sulfate), 200mg chromium, and 350mg magnesium daily. While also adding ½ teaspoon of nigella sativa powder twice daily. The individual taking this concoction monitored their blood sugar daily and gradually reduced their insulin intake over 6 months until her A1C levels were in a healthy range. Now she is free of diabetes and insulin shots.

What's unique about vanadium is that vanadium compounds act in an insulin-mimetic fashion both in vitro and in vivo, which has been well established. Both inorganic and organic vanadium compounds have been shown to lower plasma glucose levels, increase peripheral glucose uptake, improve insulin sensitivity, decrease plasma lipid levels, and normalize liver enzyme activities in a variety of animal models of both type I and type II diabetes.

When using chromium and vanadium, you need to figure out what exact dosage works best for you, as there is no daily RDI for either. With chromium, research has found 1000mcg daily to be a safe upper limit.

Vanadium

Vanadium (vanadyl sulfate) has been shown in research to regenerate pancreatic B-cells (insulin-producing cells) in type 1 diabetes animal models. The research article **"Vanadyl Sulfate Treatment Stimulates Proliferation and Regeneration of Beta Cells in Pancreatic Islets"** states -

"Furthermore, in the STZ-diabetic group, the decrease in the number of insulin immunopositive beta cells was corrected to reach the control level mainly with the higher dose of vanadium. Therefore, VOSO4 treatment normalized plasma glucose and insulin levels and improved insulin sensitivity in STZ-experimental diabetes and induced beta cell

proliferation and/or regeneration in normal or diabetic rats."

*STZ - STZ(Streptozotocin) damages the beta cells, which results in hyperglycemia and hypoinsulinemia. This mimics the phenotypes of Type 1 diabetes in mice.
*VOSO4 - vanadium sulfate

The article "**The role of vanadium in the management of diabetes**" states -

"recent discoveries that indicate a possible role for vanadium in management of the disease. In vitro, vanadium salts mimic most effects of insulin on the main target tissues of the hormone, and in vivo they induce a sustained fall in blood glucose levels in insulin-deficient diabetic rats, and improve glucose homeostasis in obese, insulin-resistant diabetic rodents. Recent short-term clinical trials with vanadium salts also seem promising in type II (non-insulin-dependent) diabetic patients in whom liver and peripheral insulin resistance was attenuated, indicating the therapeutic potential of vanadium salts, pending demonstration of their long-term innocuity."

The research article "**Vanadium and diabetes**" states -

"We demonstrated in 1985 that vanadium administered in the drinking water to streptozotocin (STZ) diabetic rats restored elevated blood glucose to normal. Subsequent studies have shown that vanadyl sulfate can lower elevated blood glucose, cholesterol and triglycerides in a variety of diabetic models including the STZ diabetic rat, the Zucker fatty rat and the Zucker diabetic fatty rat. Long-term studies of up to one year did not show toxicity in control or STZ rats administered vanadyl sulfate in doses that lowered elevated blood glucose. In the BB diabetic rat, a model of insulin-dependent diabetes, vanadyl sulfate lowered the insulin requirement by up to 75%. Vanadyl sulfate is effective orally when administered by either single dose or chronic doses. It is also effective by the intraperitoneal route. We have also been able to demonstrate marked long-term effects of vanadyl sulfate in diabetic animals following treatment and withdrawal of vanadyl sulfate."

The research article "**Long- term efficacy and safety of vanadium in the treatment of type 1 diabetes**" states -

"Background: Vanadium compounds are able to reduce blood glucose in experimentally- induced diabetic rats and type 2 diabetic patients, but data about their long- term safety and efficacy in diabetic patients are scarce.

Methods: Fourteen type 1 diabetic patients received oral vanadyl sulfate (50 - 100 mg TID) for a period of 30 months. Fasting blood sugar (FBS), lipid levels, hematologic, and biochemical parameters were measured before and periodically during the treatment.

Results: The daily doses of insulin decreased from 37.2 ± 5.5 to 25.8 ± 17.3 units/day and at the same time the mean FBS decreased from 238 ± 71 to 152 ± 42 mg/dL. Meanwhile, there was a decrease in plasma total cholesterol without any change in triglyceride level. No significant clinical or paraclinical side effects, with the exception for mild diarrhea at the beginning of treatment, were observed during 30 months therapy.

*TID: ter in die: three times a day
*three capsules of 75 – 100 mg vanadyl; equivalent to 1.5 mg elemental vanadium/kg/day)

Chromium

Chromium is an essential mineral necessary for normal glucose and lipid homeostasis. Severe chromium deficiency is known to cause reversible insulin resistance and diabetes.

Trivalent chromium in a complex known as glucose tolerance factor is considered the biologically active form. Chromium chloride, chromium nicotinate, and chromium picolinate are commonly used formulations of trivalent chromium. Chromium picolinate is considered the most effective form of chromium supplementation, and doses of 200–1,000 mcg per day have been shown to improve blood glucose control.

According to the American IOM (Institute of Medicine), following an extensive review of scientific literature about chromium picolinate, there is no reason to set an upper limit (UL) for Chromium.

In theory, this means there are no substantive safety concerns about chromium.
See Chapter 4 "Insulin Resistance" for more information on chromium.

Nigella Sativa

Powdered nigella sativa seeds have shown incredible efficacy in animal and human models in stimulating pancreatic B-cells to release insulin and B-cell proliferation.

The research article "**Mechanism of the antidiabetic action of Nigella sativa and Thymoquinone: a review**" states-

"Long used in traditional medicine, Nigella sativa (NS; Ranunculaceae) has shown significant efficacy as an adjuvant therapy for diabetes mellitus (DM) management by improving glucose tolerance, decreasing hepatic gluconeogenesis, normalizing blood sugar and lipid imbalance, and stimulating insulin secretion from pancreatic cells".

The research article "**Nigella sativa Oil Has Significant Repairing Ability of Damaged Pancreatic Tissue Occurs in Induced Type 1 Diabetes Mellitus**" states-

"Type 1 diabetes mellitus (T1DM) is a chronic autoimmune disease that impairs production of insulin. The disruption of insulin synthesis is caused by an autoimmune destruction of pancreatic islet

cells. Nigella sativa oil (NSO) was known as hypoglycemic agent in both types of diabetes but little known about its ability of repairing the pancreatic damage occurred in T1DM. By intraperitoneal injection of a single dose of streptozotocin (STZ) (65 mg/kg), T1DM was induced in overnight fasted 24 rats. They were equally divided into four groups as following; (1) control group; (2) diabetic non treated group, (3) and (4) groups were treated with different doses of NSO (0.2 and 0.4 ml/kg) respectively, for a period of 30 consecutive days. Blood glucose was tested every morning through the experimental period. After completion the experimental protocol, blood samples were collected and serum insulin was assayed using ELISA. The pancreatic tail was dissected and kept in 10% formalin. The samples were processed using a tissue processor for histological study after H and E staining. The control group showed normal cells in pancreatic islet of Langerhans. The diabetic group with no treatment showed shrunken islets of Langerhans displaying degenerative and necrotic changes. Meanwhile, the treatment with low dose NSO protected the majority of cells in the islet of Langerhans, however the high dose NSO treatment showed a similar morphology as in normal control group (GA), so that resulted in significant elevation *of serum insulin level (p<0.005). The data suggests that NSO treatment has a therapeutic effect against STZ induced T1DM rats.*

In the article "**Antidiabetic Properties of a Spice Plant Nigella sativa**" states-

"Kanter and co-workers have studied effect of N. sativa on streptozotocin (STZ) induced diabetes in rats. Diabetes was induced in rats by a single intraperitoneal injection of STZ (50 mg/kg). The animals became diabetic within 24 hours after the administration of STZ. Intraperitoneal injection of 0.20 ml/kg volatile oil of N. Sativa seeds for 30 days in such rats, caused gradual partial regeneration/proliferation of pancreatic beta-cells, decrease in the elevated serum glucose and increase of the lowered serum insulin concentrations .

What if I need an amputation due to infection?

I had a client with a thumb infection that required amputation. She had consulted me on what she could do. So I immediately asked her if she was diabetic, and she confirmed that she had type 2 diabetes.

So I explained to her that whether she used pharmaceuticals or natural antimicrobials for the infection, she needed a functioning immune system. The reason why people with HIV die is HIV destroys their immune system enabling regular infections to become fatal. Without a somewhat functioning immune system, antimicrobials cannot work properly. High blood sugar, or hyperglycemia, can stress the body and make it harder for the immune system's white blood cells to function, weakening the immune system and making it less effective. This can make people with diabetes more susceptible to infections.

So I told her first to take 350mg of magnesium glycinate and 200mcg of chromium daily to control her blood sugar. I also told her to take ½ teaspoon of powdered black seeds(nigella sativa) twice daily. After five days, I told her to take 6 drops of prediluted oregano oil(origanum vulgare) under the tongue every day until the infection subsided.

Her thumb healed within two weeks and no longer needed to be amputated.

Chapter 5

A List of Antidiabetic & Blood Sugar Reducing
Foods, Spices & Herbs

Bitter melon (Momordica charantia)
Bitter Albott (Neurolaena lobata)
Cerasee (Momordica balsamimna)
Jack Ina Bush (Chromolaena odorata)
Soursop (Annona muricata)
Ceylon Cinnamon (Cinnamomum verum)
Spiny Amaranth (Amaranthus spinosus)
Pendant Amaranth (Amaranthus caudatus)
Berberine
Oil of Oregano(Origanum vulgare)
Ginger(Zingiber officinale Roscoe)
Fenugreek(Trigonella foenum-graceum)
Ginseng(Panax Ginseng)
Rosemary(Rosmarinus officinalis L.)
Eryngium longifolium
Rhizome of Alsophila firma
Nopal/Prickly pear cactus (Opuntia ficus-indica)
Gymnema/Gurmar (Gymnema sylvestre)
Turmeric(Curcuma longa)
Mango Leaf(Mangifera Indica)
Neem(Azadirachta indica)
Jamun Seed(Syzygium cumini)
Curry Leaves(Murraya koenigii)

Aloe Juice(Aloe barbadensis miller)

Bibliography

Environmental Chemicals and Type 2 Diabetes: An Updated Systematic Review of the Epidemiologic Evidence

Chin-Chi Kuo, MD, MPH,1,2,3 Katherine Moon, MPH,1,2,3 Kristina A. Thayer, PhD,4 and Ana Navas-Acien, MD, PhD

Impact of Glyphosate on the Development of Insulin Resistance in Experimental Diabetic Rats: Role of NFκB Signalling Pathways

Monisha Prasad, Methodology, Mansour K. Gatasheh, Mohammad A. Alshuniaber,3 Rajapandiyan Krishnamoorthy

Does Vitamin D Have a Role in Diabetes?

Monitoring Editor: Alexander Muacevic and John R Adler
Tahani M Abugoukh, Afrah Al Sharaby, Abeer O Elshaikh, Malaz Joda Amna Madni, Ihab Ahmed, Rasha S Abdalla Kholood Ahmed Shahd E Elazrag, and Nadir Abdelrahman

A scientific review: the role of chromium in insulin resistance

Peter J Havel

Magnesium and type 2 diabetes

Mario Barbagallo and Ligia J Dominguez

Why does obesity cause diabetes?

Samuel Klein , Amalia Gastaldelli , Hannele Yki-Järvinen , Philipp E Scherer

Does physical activity modify the risk of obesity for type 2 diabetes: a review of epidemiological data

Li Qin, Mirjam J. Knol, Eva Corpeleijn, and Ronald P. Stolk

Vanadium compounds as insulin mimics
C Orvig, K H Thompson, M Battell, J H McNeill

Mechanism of the antidiabetic action of Nigella sativa and Thymoquinone: a review
Arslan Shaukat, Arsalan Zaidi, Haseeb Anwar, and Nadeem Kizilbash

Antidiabetic Properties of a Spice Plant Nigella sativa
Murli L. Mathur, Jyoti Gaur, Ruchika Sharma, Kripa Ram Haldiya

Insulin Resistance
Andrew M. Freeman; Luis A. Acevedo; Nicholas Pennings

Mapping the global research landscape on insulin resistance: Visualization and bibliometric analysis
Sa'ed H Zyoud, Muna Shakhshir, Amer Koni, Amani S Abushanab, Moyad Shahwan, Ammar Abdulrahman Jairoun, Rand Al Subu, Adham Abu Taha, and Samah W Al-Jabi

Obesity, Insulin Resistance, and Type 2 Diabetes: Associations and Therapeutic Implications
Yohannes Tsegyie Wondmkun

Vitamin D deficiency and diabetes

Medicinal plants of India with anti-diabetic potential
J K Grover, S Yadav, V Vats

Medicinal plants and phytochemicals with anti-obesogenic potentials: A review
Ramgopal Mopuri , Md Shahidul Islam

Cocoa: a functional food that decreases insulin resistance and oxidative damage in young adults with class II obesity

José Arnold González-Garrido, José Rubén García-Sánchez, Carlos Javier López-Victorio, Adelma Escobar-Ramírez, and Ivonne María Olivares-Corichi

Cocoa flavanols show beneficial effects in cultured pancreatic beta cells and liver cells to prevent the onset of type 2 diabetes

María Ángeles Martín, Isabel Cordero-Herrera, Laura Bravo, Sonia Ramos, Luis Goya

Monomeric cocoa catechins enhance β-cell function by increasing mitochondrial respiration

Thomas J. Rowley IV a, Benjamin F. Bitner, Jason D. Ray a, Daniel R. Lathen, Andrew T. Smithson, Blake W. Dallon, Chase J. Plowman, Benjamin T. Bikman b, Jason M. Hansen, Melanie R. Dorenkott, Katheryn M. Goodrich, Liyun Ye, Sean F. O'Keefe, Andrew P. Neilson, Jeffery S. Tessem

Dietary Flavonol Epicatechin Prevents the Onset of Type 1 Diabetes in Non-obese Diabetic (NOD) Mice

Zhuo Fu, Julia Yuskavage, and Dongmin Liu

Acknowledgments

I thank my great ancestral spirits for guiding my pen in writing this life-changing treatise. I thank The great Goddess Asase Ya for providing the healing plants that we the children of the earth can use to heal and repair our bodies. I thank the great permeating all-encompassing life force, Onyankopon, for my intelligence and ability to expose this healing knowledge to the world.

Sean Martu

Made in the USA
Middletown, DE
22 August 2024

58975554R00035